Dash Diet

Comprehensive 21-day Dash Diet Meal Plan, Valuable Strategies For Reducing Sodium Intake, And Nutritious Recipes For Promoting Healthy Eating Habits In Both Professional And Residential Environments

Alexander Grewal

TABLE OF CONTENT

Introduction

The purpose of this cookbook is to provide easily prepared DASH diet recipes that are straightforward to grasp. Over the past decade, the adoption of the DASH diet strategy has witnessed a steady rise among a growing number of individuals. The Dietary Approaches to Stop Hypertension (referred to as the DASH) diet is gaining prominence as a growing number of individuals acknowledge its efficacy in managing hypertension and elevated blood glucose levels. The DASH diet frequently incorporates meals rich in potassium, calcium, and magnesium, while maintaining a low sodium content. The dietary guidelines also restrict the consumption of carbonated beverages, refined carbohydrates, and sugar.

In light of contemporary lifestyles, experiencing fatigue and succumbing to an unhealthy dietary regimen is highly atypical. Consequently, there has been a surge in the prevalence of diabetes and blood sugar disorders among the younger population. Cardiac problems previously detected in the elderly demographic have now manifested themselves in individuals in their early thirties. The imperative to uncover strategies for regaining a state of well-being has been significantly intensified. Consequently, numerous individuals intend to employ the DASH diet as a modality for addressing said disorders. This culinary guide serves as an optimum resource for effectively managing elevated blood sugar levels and hypertension.

The creation of this cookbook is the result of rigorous research, which allowed us to concentrate on recipes that are uncomplicated to make and utilize ingredients that are easily obtainable in the kitchen.

The objective of the book is not only to provide guidance to experienced individuals but also to aid those with less expertise in effectively executing the recipes, which are presented in a concise and easily comprehensible fashion. The book features an extensive repast spanning a period of 21 days. This comprehensive package includes breakfast, lunch, and dinner meals to assist you in managing the entirety of the month.

The meal plan outlined in the book has been carefully crafted, taking into consideration the busy lifestyles of individuals The meals are designed in accordance with the body's daily dietary requirements, guaranteeing the inclusion of all essential nutrients. The meal plan enables you to monitor your advancement and regulate your dietary intake. If you engage the services of a personal chef, they will simply adhere to the designated meal plan, ensuring your peace of mind by alleviating the responsibility of caloric calculations.

Individuals who are incapable of engaging in routine culinary tasks could potentially prepare excessive amounts of food and subsequently store it in the refrigerator. Not only will this be a time-saving measure, but it will also help you adhere to your dietary regimen. Additionally, the reader has the opportunity to strategically plan and organize meals at their convenience.

Consideration and effort have been invested in curating a compilation of culinary instructions that not only facilitate the regulation of your calorie consumption, but also ensure that the delectable essence of each dish remains uncompromised. Individuals who seek to regulate their blood glucose levels frequently prioritize the consumption of bland and flavorless food items. Although some individuals are capable of sustaining such a practice, the majority of individuals relinquish it due to a deficiency in taste. The recipes encompassed within the book serve the dual purpose of enhancing your well-being while affording you the opportunity to explore novel culinary traditions.

The recipes featured in this book offer a novel approach to managing your blood sugar levels, providing you with the opportunity to derive satisfaction from the entire process.

The DASH Diet

With an increasing number of individuals experiencing illnesses related to high blood pressure, the DASH diet offers a unique treatment option that has been duly validated through scientific and clinical experimentation. In the course of the last decade, there has been a noteworthy surge in the prevalence of hypertension, affecting more than one billion individuals worldwide who are grappling with ailments associated with elevated blood pressure. Because of this steady increase, the DASH diet has become one of the most efficient ways to cope with the condition.

Could you please provide a precise explanation of the DASH diet?

The Dietary Approaches to Stop Hypertension (DASH) dietary regimen, which has received the endorsement of the National Heart, Lung, and Blood

Institute in the United States, examines the nutritional composition of food to devise distinct dietary patterns that aid in the reduction of elevated blood pressure levels. The dietary regimen has been developed as a result of collaborative efforts between bio-scientists and legislators, aimed at identifying the constituents of an individual's diet that need to be eliminated for the purpose of controlling increases in blood pressure.

The development of the DASH diet was prompted by the observed surge in the prevalence of hypertension among individuals over the course of the past two decades. As a consequence of this, healthcare experts, in partnership with the United States Department of Health and Human Services, took initiative to devise approaches aimed at managing hypertension and mitigating the multitude of risks associated with elevated blood pressure. After an extensive investigation, the researchers made the observation that individuals who consumed a greater quantity of vegetables or adhered to a diet predominantly composed of plant-based foods exhibited a reduced incidence of elevated blood pressure indicators and instances. Consequently, this established the fundamental basis of the DASH diet.

The DASH diet places an emphasis on the ingestion of unprocessed and predominantly organic constituents. This dietary approach places significant emphasis on the consumption of whole grains, fruits, vegetables, and lean meats. In severe instances, individuals displaying noticeable symptoms of heart-related illnesses due to elevated blood pressure are recommended to adopt a vegan diet for a certain duration, aiming to mitigate complications associated with hypertension.

The dietary regimen also mandates the complete avoidance of sodium. Due to the adverse effects of excessive salt and oil intake on blood pressure regulation within the human body, the dietary guidelines of the DASH diet significantly restrict the consumption of salt. The DASH diet meals consist of a nutritious combination of leafy greens, low-fat proteins, and unrefined grains.

Optimal selections would include unprocessed fruits, low-fat dairy items, and lean sources of protein like poultry, fish, and a diverse range of legumes. In addition to reducing salt intake, it is advisable to refrain from consuming foods rich in red meat, refined carbohydrates, and saturated fat. According to conventional practice, individuals adhering to the DASH diet should avoid consuming quantities of salt exceeding 1 teaspoon (equivalent to 2,300 mg) per day.

The diet is deemed secure for adherence and has received official endorsement by the US Department of Agriculture (USDA). The DASH diet, alongside two other healthful diets, was featured in the 2015-2020 US Dietary Guidelines.

The History Of The Dash Diet

Over the past several years, there has been a notable rise in the prevalence of hypertension or elevated blood pressure among individuals.

Researchers have determined that the foremost determinant contributing to the emergence of the condition is an unfavorable lifestyle, predominantly characterized by an unwholesome dietary regimen. To effectively control and mitigate hypertension, it is imperative to adhere to a nourishing dietary regimen.

The DASH diet is a well-established dietary approach utilized for the purpose of managing hypertension. It has been derived from empirical data generated through meticulous research undertaken by distinguished professionals in the realm of medical science. Numerous individuals are presently adhering to the dietary regimen prescribed by their medical practitioners in order to attain regulated levels of blood pressure.

However, have you ever pondered upon the origins and historical background of the DASH Diet? In order to fully understand how the diet works, you must know its beginning and history.

The Origins and Historical Development of the DASH Diet

The diet has been devised in response to the rising prevalence of hypertension among individuals, as indicated by statistical analyses. It is crucial to mitigate the elevation of blood pressure as it has a strong correlation with the onset of severe cardiovascular ailments such as congestive heart failure, myocardial infarction, and various other afflictions. Given that it has been ascertained that the diet plays a significant role in the onset of hypertension, researchers have devised the Dietary Approaches to Stop Hypertension (DASH) diet as a means of managing the condition.

"DASH" represents the abbreviation of Dietary Approaches to Halt Hypertension. The investigations pertaining to the dietary aspects were initiated in 1992 and were carried out at five esteemed global research institutions. The primary objective of the studies was to establish the impact of dietary factors on hypertension. Upon comprehending the correlation between blood pressure and diet as evidenced by experimental studies and tests, the concept of the DASH diet was formulated.

The researchers employed three dietary regimens in order to ascertain the most suitable diet. Two of the diets were considered as independent variables in the study, whereas the remaining diet was designated as the control. The control diet comprises the typical dietary regimen prevalent among the majority of individuals.

The initial experimental regimen is the "diet emphasizing fruits and vegetables," where the quantity of fruits and vegetables has been augmented along with a subsequent elevation in magnesium and potassium mineral content.

The second experimental dietary intervention consists of a reduced fat content, elevated levels of fiber, potassium, magnesium, calcium, and protein. The research was undertaken with a sample size of 459 individuals hailing from diverse global regions.

Based on extensive experimentation and thorough analysis of the collected data, it has been determined that the second experimental diet is the most efficacious iteration of the DASH diet.

The present dietary regimen being employed, known as the DASH diet, encompasses the ensuing categories of food groups:

-grains

-vegetables

-fruits

-meat, poultry, fish

-low-fat dairy products

-seeds

-oils

-sweets

It is recommended that hypertensive individuals consume controlled portions of these foods as part of their diet to help reduce blood pressure.

Additionally, recent studies have elucidated that the DASH diet is efficacious in the reduction of blood cholesterol levels, which serves as a contributing element to cardiovascular disorders. It is also under investigation to determine its impact on facilitating weight reduction and mitigating the risk of various types of cancers.

The DASH diet stands out as one of the most extensively studied dietary approaches in history. There is no need for you to harbor any reservations regarding the meal program, as it is exclusively comprised of organic, safe, and nutritious offerings. It is highly advised to not only manage hypertension but also to take proactive measures to prevent its occurrence.

Frequently Asked Questions (F.A.Q)

Q. Does the DASH platform offer individualized medical guidance?

No, it does not. Whilst a collaborative effort by a team of dietitians and doctors culminated in the development of the DASH diet, it should be noted that it cannot serve as a substitute for the individualized healthcare delivered by your physician. It is highly recommended that you continue to place your trust in the guidance provided by your physician for the purposes of receiving personalized medical care.

Nevertheless, the DASH diet does offer a balanced and nutritionally adequate eating plan in accordance with overarching dietary recommendations. Furthermore, the American Heart Association endorses this diet and it aligns with health recommendations and guidelines endorsed globally. If you possess a particular concern arising from your individual requirements, it is advisable to engage in a conversation about this dietary regimen with a personal medical practitioner.

Q. Are there any recommendations for physical activity given alongside this dietary plan?

The core foundation of the DASH diet rests predominantly on the principles of nutrition. Nonetheless, individuals adhering to this dietary regimen are advised to additionally adhere to the customary protocols of engaging in physical activity for a duration of 30 minutes on the majority of days in a week. If weight loss is your objective, the DASH diet suggests a minimum of 60 minutes of daily exercise to be incorporated into your routine.

Q. Might I inquire if it is permissible for me to follow this particular diet plan given my dietary adherence to vegetarianism?

Indeed, the DASH diet can readily be tailored to accommodate a vegetarian dietary pattern. The DASH diet was initially developed with reference to a vegetarian diet, as it was observed that individuals following vegetarianism exhibited a propensity for reduced blood pressure levels. The dietary regimen employed in the study that showcased the efficacy of the DASH diet did indeed encompass animal protein sources, including but not limited to meat, fish, and dairy products. Nevertheless, comparable advantages can be acquired through the utilization of plant-based protein sources.

Please bear in mind that the DASH diet consists of a diverse range of fruits and vegetables, low-fat dairy products, and restricted consumption of fats and oils. The aforementioned suggestions apply universally to individuals adhering to a vegetarian diet. To fulfill your DASH dietary objectives for meats, we suggest replacing meat portions with nuts, seeds, and legumes.

Q. May I inquire about the efficacy of this diet?

The investigation conducted on the DASH diet revealed that individuals with pre-hypertension who adhered to this dietary regimen observed a noteworthy decrease in blood pressure ranging from 3 to 6 mm Hg. Similarly, those who already had hypertension experienced a reduction ranging from 6 to 11 mm Hg. Remarkably, these reductions were observed without any associated alterations in body weight.

Q. What is the extent of salt restriction?

There exist two distinct variations of the DASH diet. The prescribed DASH diet permits an individual to ingest a maximum of 2,300 milligrams of sodium per day. The low sodium DASH diet is characterized by greater restrictiveness and advocates for a daily consumption of no more than 1,500 milligrams. In individuals with sensitivity to sodium, its intake has the potential to elevate blood pressure. If the conventional diet fails to yield desired results, adoption of the DASH diet with reduced sodium may be considered.

Both dietary interventions have been demonstrated to cause a substantial decrease in blood pressure levels among individuals. The contemporary dietary intake encompasses approximately 3,500 milligrams of sodium. Research has indicated that reducing sodium intake yields a favorable impact on blood pressure, particularly among individuals aged 40 and above.

Q. Can I expect to experience weight reduction while adhering to this specific dietary plan?

The DASH diet was not formulated with the primary objective of facilitating weight loss. The primary objective was to decrease blood pressure. Nevertheless, this dietary plan is conducive to maintaining good health and can be employed as an effective means of achieving weight loss. In adherence to the conventional DASH diet, an individual is granted the privilege of consuming a maximum of five portions of sugary treats on a weekly basis. Nevertheless, if your objective is to attain weight loss, it is advisable to decrease or entirely remove the consumption of these sugary treats. Additionally, you have the option to select a DASH diet plan that offers a caloric intake lower than what is required for gradual weight loss. While the conventional DASH diet prescribes a daily calorie intake of 2,000, alternatives of 1,800 or 1,600 calories are selectable.

Q. Can you please elaborate on additional advantages associated with adhering to the DASH dietary approach?

This diet has received a significantly high endorsement from medical professionals. The diet recommended by the Mayo Clinic is suitable for individuals of average constitution due to its provision of an optimal combination of essential nutrients. Moreover, this diet might additionally contribute to safeguarding against conditions such as stroke, cancer, cardiovascular ailments, diabetes, and osteoporosis.

Q. What specific food items are permitted and prohibited according to the guidelines of this dietary plan?

There are no foods that are strictly prohibited on this dietary plan. Nevertheless, it is advisable to anticipate a substantial intake of fruits, vegetables, reduced-fat dairy, whole grain products, and also incorporate legumes, poultry, and fish into your diet. The food items that are restricted within the DASH diet include red meat, fatty substances, and sugary treats. It exhibits notably low levels of saturated fat, overall fat content, and cholesterol. It is advisable to restrict the consumption of processed foods as a general principle. Rather, it is advisable that you cook your own meals at home as a means of minimizing the consumption of sodium.

Q. Is it permissible for me to dine outside while adhering to my dietary restrictions?

Indeed, there is no need for you to impose limitations on yourself when it comes to dining at restaurants. In order to foster adherence to the DASH diet, it is recommended to seek out dining establishments that feature a selection of freshly sourced fruits and vegetables, accompanied by cuisine that is prepared with reduced fat content. Numerous dining establishments offer a variety of heart-healthy alternatives, which you might consider opting for. If you will be dining at an upscale establishment, you have the option to inquire with your server regarding menu items that are low in sodium and fat, or kindly request the chef to customize your meal without the addition of salt.

Q. What techniques can I employ to enhance the flavor in culinary preparations?

There is a wide array of alternatives available to enhance the taste of your food while simultaneously reducing your reliance on sodium. Select fresh herbs and spices that are replete with flavorful attributes and will not contribute to your overall sodium consumption. An alternative option would be to select seasonings with reduced sodium content, such as Mrs. DASH seasoning blends. Please check the selection of your local grocery store for potassium salt, which is sometimes referred to as lite salt. The majority of individuals experience a shift in their taste preferences as they age, leading them to no longer have an inclination towards dishes with a high sodium content. While modest quantities of salt may still be permissible, it is advisable to refrain from excessive consumption at all times.

Q. What additional advantages can I expect to observe?

Although the DASH diet does not explicitly advocate for any other advantages, you may observe an improvement in both your physical appearance and overall well-being on a regular basis. By enhancing your consumption of fruits and vegetables, you are likely to obtain a higher proportion of vital vitamins and minerals within your dietary intake. Numerous individuals attest to experiencing heightened levels of energy on a daily basis. Should your present dietary regimen not align with the tenets of the DASH diet, anticipate more significant alterations upon adopting this particular dietary approach.

Fundamentals of the DASH Diet for Novice Individuals

The Dash diet has garnered endorsement from numerous esteemed health institutes, such as the U.S. Department of Agriculture, which advocates for the universal adoption of the Dash diet as the optimal and beneficial dietary regimen for all Americans. According to official statements from the National Institutes of Health, the Dash diet not only promotes the cultivation of wholesome dietary habits, but also provides recommendations on nutritious alternatives to processed and unhealthy food items.

The proponents of the Dash diet have asserted that in addition to its objective of reducing hypertension, this dietary approach also aids individuals in reducing their sodium (salt) intake while simultaneously augmenting their potassium, magnesium, and calcium consumption.

Key attributes of the Dash diet comprise:

Lowers sodium intake

Decrease in the consumption of alcohol and caffeine.

Increased fiber consumption

Augmented consumption of beneficial fats

Increased vitamins and minerals

Individualized sodium and caloric consumption.

Within the framework of the Dash diet, individuals have the option to follow a daily caloric intake ranging from 1500 to 3100 calories. Additionally, you have the option to select either a 2300mg/day or a 1500 mg/day sodium intake Dash diet.

The determination of your suitable calorie intake is contingent upon various factors such as your level of physical activity, body weight, as well as the presence or prevention of high blood pressure.

If an individual is grappling with excess weight, it is probable that they will opt for the lower calorie intake threshold. If you maintain an active lifestyle, it is probable that you will opt for the higher caloric intake level.

If you are afflicted with hypertension or are susceptible to its onset due to familial predisposition, and so on. In that case, it is advisable to opt for a low sodium diet.

It would be advisable for you to collaborate with your healthcare professional in order to establish an appropriate calorie and sodium intake regimen that aligns with your individual needs.

Minimization of caffeine and alcohol consumption

The Dash diet recommends restricting the consumption of tea, coffee, alcoholic beverages, and carbonated beverages. They provide negligible nutritional benefits; generally, they are high in refined sugars and have the potential to raise blood pressure levels.

Increased fiber consumption

The Dash diet advises individuals to enhance their fiber intake by regularly consuming multiple servings of fruits, vegetables, and grains on a daily basis. Engaging in this practice will contribute to a heightened sense of satiety and aid in the reduction of blood pressure levels.

The consumption of substantial amounts of dietary fiber additionally aids in the regulation of blood glucose levels and promotes the process of weight reduction.

Increased good fats

The Dash diet advocates for the consumption of substantial amounts of healthy fats while reducing the intake of unhealthy fats. It is recommended to substitute Trans fats and Saturated fats with omega-3 fatty acids sourced from fish and seafood, low-fat dairy products, nuts, seeds, and lean cuts of meat.

When individuals incorporate beneficial fats into their diet, it can effectively contribute to enhancing their overall well-being, as these fats have the potential to decrease levels of unhealthy cholesterol while simultaneously raising levels of beneficial cholesterol.

Increased vitamins & minerals

On the Dash diet, an assortment of fruits, vegetables, whole grains, and other recommended foods will furnish you with vital vitamins and minerals.

Veggie Scramble

Ingredients

- 6 white button mushrooms, sliced
- 1/2 teaspoon salt substitute
- 1/2 teaspoon freshly ground pepper
- 6 egg whites
- 1/4 cup fresh parsley, chopped

- 1 teaspoon olive oil
- 1/2 large red bell pepper, julienned
- 1/2 large yellow pepper, julienned
- 1 small sweet white onion, chopped
- 1 clove garlic, crushed

Preparation

In a generously-sized and weighty skillet, elevate the heat to medium-high and proceed to warm the olive oil. Incorporate peppers, onion, and garlic into the mixture, and proceed to sauté them for approximately 5 minutes until the vegetables reach a state of tender-crisp texture. Incorporate mushrooms into the mixture and cook over medium heat for an additional 2 minutes.

Incorporate salt alternative and freshly cracked pepper into the egg whites, then proceed to transfer the mixture into the skillet. Cook the eggs until they reach the desired level of doneness, taking care not to overcook them. Complete the presentation by adding a sprinkling of fresh parsley as a garnish, and offer the dish either on its own or accompanied by a slice of whole-grain toast.

American Blueberry Pancakes

Ingredients

- 150g pack blueberries
- sunflower oil or a little butter for cooking
- golden or maple syrup
- 200g self-raising flour
- 1 tsp baking powder
- 1 egg
- 300ml milk
- knob butter

Directions

Combine the flour, baking powder, and a small amount of salt in a spacious bowl. Whisk together the beaten egg and milk, then create a hollow in the middle of the dry ingredients. Gradually incorporate the milk into the mixture, whisking diligently until a thick, silky batter is formed. Incorporate the melted butter by beating it in, and delicately fold in half of the blueberries.

Warm a teaspoon of oil or a small piece of butter in a spacious non-stick skillet. Place a generous tablespoon of the batter per pancake onto the pan to form pancakes with a diameter of approximately 7.5cm. Prepare three to four pancakes concurrently. Cook for approximately three minutes over a moderate heat until small bubbles become visible on the surface of each pancake, then flip and cook for an additional two to three minutes until they achieve a golden hue. Place a layer of kitchen paper over the pancakes to preserve their warmth while you finish using the remaining batter. Accompany with a drizzle of golden syrup along with the remaining fresh blueberries.

Spinach And Egg Breakfast Muffins

- ½ cup roasted red pepper, chopped
- 2 oz. prosciutto, chopped
- ½ cup skim milk
- Cooking spray as needed
- 1 cup (low-fat variety) cheese, crumbled
- 4 oz. spinach, chopped
- 6 eggs

1.
    In a mixing bowl, thoroughly mix the eggs, milk, cheese, spinach, red pepper, and prosciutto.
2. Grease the muffin tins with some cooking spray.
3. Pour the muffin mix in the tins.
4. Bake in the preheated oven at 350 degrees F for 25-30 minutes.
5. Serve warm.

Over the recent years, there has been a noticeable upward trend in the prevalence of hypertension or elevated blood pressure among individuals.

Scholars have ascertained that the paramount determinant leading to the onset of the affliction is an unhealthy way of life, predominantly characterized by an unhealthy dietary regime. To effectively manage and mitigate hypertension, it is of utmost importance to adhere to a nutritious dietary regimen.

The DASH diet is regarded as one of the most well-established dietary approaches utilized for the purpose of managing hypertension. It has been derived from scientific studies conducted by medical experts in the field. A considerable number of individuals are presently adopting the dietary plan endorsed by their medical practitioners to attain and maintain optimal blood pressure levels.

Have you ever pondered the origins and historical development of the DASH Diet? To acquire a comprehensive comprehension of the diet's functioning, one must possess knowledge pertaining to its inception and historical evolution.

The Commencement and Historical Background of the DASH Diet

The dietary plan has been devised in response to the rising prevalence of hypertension among individuals, as revealed by meticulous statistical analyses. It is of utmost significance to mitigate the rise in blood pressure, as it is closely linked to the progression of severe cardiovascular ailments, encompassing heart failure, myocardial infarction, and numerous other afflictions. In view of the fact that diet plays a substantial role in the onset of hypertension, researchers have devised the DASH diet as a means to effectively regulate the condition.

"DASH" stands for Dietary Approaches to Stop Hypertension, representing a set of dietary guidelines specifically designed to mitigate the effects of high blood pressure. The investigations pertaining to the diet commenced in 1992 and were carried out across five esteemed global research institutions.

The primary objective of the investigations was to determine the impact of dietary factors on hypertension. Upon comprehending the pivotal role of diet in influencing blood pressure through rigorous experimentation and examination of the subjects, the notion of the DASH diet was formulated.

The researchers utilized three distinct diets to ascertain the most suitable dietary regimen. Two of the diets were considered independent variables, whereas the remaining diet functioned as the control group. The control diet encompasses the conventional dietary habits predominantly observed among the general population.

The initial experimental dietary intervention involves adopting a "fruits and vegetables diet," wherein there has been a deliberate augmentation in the intake of fruits and vegetables, leading to an elevation in magnesium and potassium mineral levels.

The second experimental diet entails a composition characterized by low-fat content, increased fiber, elevated levels of potassium, magnesium, and calcium, as well as a heightened protein quantity. The research trials were carried out on a sample group consisting of 459 individuals hailing from diverse geographic regions across the globe.

Based on extensive experimentation and meticulous analysis of the gathered data, it has been determined that the second experimental diet is the most efficacious among all DASH diets.

The present dietary regimen in use is comprised of the subsequent categorizations of food:

-grains

-vegetables

-fruits

-meat, poultry, fish

-low-fat dairy products

-seeds

-oils

-sweets

These food items should be consumed in controlled quantities by individuals with hypertension as a means of assisting in the reduction of blood pressure.

Subsequent research has also unveiled that the DASH diet exhibits efficacy in reducing blood cholesterol levels, which is a contributing element to cardiovascular ailments. Furthermore, extensive research is currently being conducted to determine the impact of this substance on facilitating weight reduction and its potential to hinder the development of various types of cancer.

The DASH diet has been extensively studied, making it one of the most extensively researched dietary approaches to date. There is no justification for harboring any doubts regarding the meal program, as it is both organic and guarantees safety and optimal nutrition. It is both advisable to actively control hypertension and to take measures for its prevention.

Cranberry-Walnut Oatmeal

Ingredients

- 2 cups water
- 4 tsp walnuts (chopped)
- 4 tsp firmly packed brown sugar
- 1 cup steel-cut oats
- 1/3 cup sweetened dried cranberries
- 1/4 tsp salt
- 1/4 tsp cinnamon (ground)

Directions:

Combine the cranberries, oats, and cinnamon in a medium-sized saucepan, then add 2 cups of water and season with a pinch of salt. Allow the mixture to cook at a high temperature. Once the mixture begins to bubble, decrease the heat to a low setting and allow it to simmer for approximately 20 minutes, until the oats have achieved a softened consistency.

Transfer the oatmeal into the serving bowls and evenly distribute 1 teaspoon of the walnuts and 1 teaspoon of the brown sugar on top. Serve immediately and enjoy.

Cauliflower Au Gratin

Ingredients:

1 cup of tea, grated Parmesan cheese
2 tbsp, well filled with breadcrumbs
1 Cauliflower
2 tbsp of claybom
Water
Milk
Salt

Method Of Preparation:

Segment the cauliflower into florets, thoroughly rinse them, and simmer gently in a mixture consisting of equal portions of milk and water, seasoned with a modest amount of salt. Apply a layer of claybom to coat the surface of the pyrex. Please place the cauliflower branches on the surface. Gently pour a layer of liquefied claybom over the surface, generously garnish with breadcrumbs, and evenly distribute the grated cheese as a final layer.

Proceed with baking for approximately ten minutes until a slight reddening appears.

The same method can be applied to produce any other variant of au gratin vegetable.

Low-Fat French Toasts

Ingredients

2 teaspoons powdered sugar
¼ teaspoon ground nutmeg
8 egg whites
¼ cup maple syrup
8 slices bread
1 teaspoon vanilla
¼ teaspoon cinnamon powder

Method

Incorporate the egg whites by vigorously stirring them in a bowl, subsequently integrating the ground nutmeg and vanilla into the mixture.

Ensure the ingredients are fully incorporated by whisking continuously.

Submerge a piece of bread into the bowl containing the mixture of beaten eggs, ensuring that both sides are uniformly coated. Proceed to evenly coat each slice of bread with the egg mixture and subsequently sprinkle cinnamon upon them.

Preheat a griddle pan over medium-high heat. Proceed by placing the slices of bread onto the pan and proceed to cook for approximately 3 minutes on each side or until a desirable golden brown color is achieved.

Arrange the French toasts neatly on a serving platter before generously dusting them with powdered sugar. Drizzle maple syrup atop the pancakes.

Serve immediately.

Baked Oatmeal

- 1/3 c. of sugar, granulated
- 2 teaspoon of vanilla
- 2 eggs or 0.5c.of lightly beaten egg substitute,
- 1/3 c. brown sugar, firmly packed
- 2 ¼ cups uncooked Old Fashioned Quaker Oats or 2 c. of Quick Quaker Oats
- ¼ teaspoon of salt
- 3 1/3 c. of milk, fat-free

Preparation:

Preheat the oven to a temperature of 176.667 degrees Celsius or 350 degrees Fahrenheit. Apply a liberal coating of cooking spray to an 8-inch square glass baking dish.

In a spacious bowl, combine rolled oats, salt, and granulated sugar.

Combine the eggs, milk, and vanilla within a standard-sized bowl and thoroughly blend the mixture. Incorporate the oat mixture thoroughly, ensuring it is well blended, before transferring it into the baking dish.

Please preheat the oven for approximately 40-45 minutes. Then, carefully remove the item from the oven and place it onto a cooling rack.

Evenly sprinkle a layer of brown sugar onto the surface of the oatmeal. Employing the reverse side of the spoon, evenly distribute the sugar to create a thin coating that covers the entire surface of the oatmeal. Return to the oven and allow the sugar to gradually dissolve for a duration of approximately 2 to 3 minutes.

Place oven to broil. Place the dish at a distance of 3 inches from the heat source and allow the sugar to caramelize and slightly bubble for a duration of approximately 1 to 2 minutes. Proceed by alternating the baking dish's position and present the dish.

Diabetes: The Dash Diet

Several dietary strategies designed to assist individuals in managing their diabetes have experienced a period of popularity, only to gradually recede into obscurity. Nevertheless, a select few have managed to retain their initial popularity. However, to be frank, what is the level of long-term efficacy these diets tend to exhibit?

The DASH diet was formulated with the objective of addressing hypertension and offering a sustainable dietary regimen featuring reduced sodium chloride content, more commonly known as table salt. Individuals suffering from diabetes have the capacity to incorporate a substantial portion of the recommended elements of the DASH diet into their eating patterns, albeit it has been scientifically proven that adhering to a vegan diet tends to yield optimal outcomes for managing diabetes.

The perplexed populace occasionally contemplates where to commence, as the catalogue of items seems to expand with each passing year. Consequently, I resolved to evaluate the prevailing diets that are presently accessible. The findings indicated that two of them exhibited notable efficacy in assisting individuals with diabetes in preserving their well-being. The DASH diet is merely one among various alternatives. Herein lies a concise overview of the knowledge I have acquired regarding this dietary regime. Prior to proceeding, let us initially examine the essential components of a nutritionally balanced diet tailored specifically for individuals with diabetes. Therefore, the following are some of these components:

Adhering to a nutritious dietary regimen entails either a restricted carbohydrate intake or incorporating a means to metabolize excess carbohydrates, such as engaging in physical activity.

Dietary fiber has imparted numerous health benefits, comprising a low glycemic index and diminished susceptibility to heart disease, diabetes, and stroke.

Low in sodium. Given the association between sodium intake and hypertension, it is imperative to eliminate its consumption.

Fat-free. In order to mitigate the risk of developing obesity, which is a known precursor to diabetes, it is often necessary to adhere to low-fat diets that primarily consist of easily metabolized carbohydrates and fats.

It is recommended that individuals with diabetes adhere to a dietary regimen that includes a potassium intake no lower than the Recommended Daily Allowance (RDA). The deleterious impact of sodium on the cardiovascular system can potentially be mitigated through the intervention of potassium, hence establishing its utmost significance.

The DASH diet possesses all of these attributes and additional ones. In addition, it possesses further attributes. Despite being tailored for individuals with diabetes, the diet has yielded comparable efficacy. It has been demonstrated to possess qualities associated with the prevention and management of diabetes, conforming to the guidelines set forth by the American Diabetes Association.

As a preventive measure, empirical evidence suggests that it aids individuals in achieving and maintaining weight loss. Due to the fact that obesity significantly increases the likelihood of developing Type 2 diabetes, this characteristic renders it an appropriate dietary choice for individuals with diabetes.

Moreover, the incorporation of the DASH diet alongside caloric restriction effectively mitigates the risk factors associated with metabolic syndrome, a medical condition that escalates the likelihood of developing diabetes. A scholarly article presented in the esteemed journal Diabetes Care in 2011 conducted research which demonstrated that individuals diagnosed with type 2 diabetes experienced notable reductions in A1C and fasting blood sugar levels after participating in an eight-week DASH trial.

Furthermore, research has demonstrated that it is more adaptable for individuals with diabetes in comparison to alternative dietary approaches, facilitating a greater level of compliance and the ability to make necessary modifications to medical guidance.

An additional benefit of this dietary regimen is its compliance with established dietary principles. This is of utmost importance, despite its seemingly trivial nature, as numerous dietary regimens impose restrictions on certain foods, thus placing individuals at risk of inadequate nutrition.

Based on an analysis of this adherence, the dietary regime aligns with the fat range advised by governmental authorities, which suggests a consumption of 20 to 35 percent of daily calories. It also remains significantly below the prescribed limit of 10 percent saturated fat, which it upholds. Proportional amounts of proteins and carbohydrates are present.

The suggested daily allowance for this mineral is contained within the recommended serving caps for salt. Individuals who identify as African-American, are above the age of 51, or have been diagnosed with conditions such as hypertension, diabetes, or chronic renal disease, are advised to adhere to a daily sodium intake restriction of 1,500 milligrams.

Potassium possesses multiple health benefits, such as its potential to mitigate the hypertensive effects of sodium, decrease the likelihood of developing renal stones, and even impede the progression of osteoporosis. This diet provides a comprehensive array of essential nutrients. This diet facilitates the consumption of fiber within the recommended daily range of 22 to 34 grams. This is quite remarkable considering the difficulties associated with obtaining the necessary daily dosage of 4,700 milligrams, which is equivalent to consuming 11 bananas on a daily basis.

For those individuals who do not attain sufficient exposure to sunlight, it is advised to consume a daily dosage of Vitamin D amounting to 15 mg. Based on the analysis of certain nutrition experts, it is suggested that the incorporation of a cereal fortified with vitamin D could potentially compensate for this deficiency.

The diet offers a suitable provision of calcium, which is imperative for the promotion of strong bones and teeth, the development of blood vessels, and the optimal performance of muscles. In accordance with governmental regulations, the recommended daily intake of 1,000-1,300 mg is effortlessly met within this particular context. 2.4 mg is the government's recommended dosage. This statement holds validity with regards to the B-12 vitamin as well.

The recommended daily intake is 6.7.

Based on the aforementioned information, it is evident that the DASH diet presents itself as an excellent choice for individuals seeking improved management of their diabetes. The diet known as "The Biggest Loser" ranks second in this aspect, yet it offers the advantage of being meticulously crafted to aid in the reduction of blood pressure, with demonstrated comparable efficacy. Hence, if you have been in pursuit of an effective dietary regimen for diabetes management, the DASH diet presents itself as a viable alternative.

Summer Fruit Salad

Ingredients:

- 2 oz low fat feta cheese, crumbled
- 1 tbsp mint leaves, thinly sliced

- 2 cups watermelon, chopped up
- 1 cup blueberries
- 2 tbsp fresh squeezed lemon juice

Directions:

1. Combine the watermelon, blueberries, and lemon juice in a bowl and mix thoroughly.
2. Add crumbled feta cheese and mint leaves over salad to serve.

The Optimal Guidance To Incorporate With The Dash Diet

If you are seeking valuable insights on the most effective approaches to achieve weight loss and sustain it in the long run, the abundance of advice available can seem daunting and perplexing.

Here are 25 valuable dietary recommendations to improve your well-being and aid in achieving weight loss.

1. Replenish your fiber intake

Dietary fiber can be sourced from nutrient-rich foods such as vegetables, organic produce, legumes, and whole grains.

Several studies have indicated that the consumption of a higher quantity of fiber-rich foods can potentially contribute to weight loss and long-term weight management.

2. Eliminate the inclusion of any excess sugar.

Added sugar, especially derived from sugary beverages, serves as a substantial contributing factor to undesirable weight gain and health conditions such as diabetes and cardiovascular diseases.

Eliminating foods that are rich in added sugars is an effective approach to reduce excessive body weight.

It is crucial to acknowledge that foods labeled as "healthy" or "natural" can indeed contain significantly high levels of sugar. Hence, it is imperative to scrutinize food labels.

3. Get ready for a diet rich in nutritious fats.

Although fat is typically the first to be reduced in efforts to slim down, incorporating nutritious fats into your diet can effectively contribute to achieving your weight loss goals.

Similarly, lipids aid in lengthening satiety, reducing cravings, and maintaining adherence to your dietary goals.

4. Minimize or reduce disturbances.

Although it may not seem detrimental to consume meals in front of your television or computer, engaging in distracted eating can lead to increased calorie consumption and weight gain.

It is recommended to retain cell phones during mealtime, as they are considered essential technological devices. Examining your online presence, correspondences, or Facebook platform elicits a level of distraction equivalent to that of television or computer usage.

5. Embark on a Path to Better Health through Walking

A number of individuals concur that they should be provided with a comprehensive exercise regimen in order to initiate their weight loss journey.

Various forms of physical activity hold importance when striving to achieve physical fitness; however, walking is an excellent and effortless method to expend calories.

In actuality, empirical evidence has demonstrated that engaging in a mere 30 minutes of daily leisurely walking can effectively contribute to weight reduction.

Moreover, it is a commendable endeavor that can be pursued both indoors and outdoors at any given time.

6. Unleash Your Culinary Potential

Preparing additional dinners at home has been observed to promote weight loss and encourage the adoption of healthier dietary habits.

Although dining out can be enjoyable and compatible with a healthy eating plan, prioritizing the preparation of home-cooked meals is an excellent approach to maintaining a stable weight.

7. Consuming a Breakfast High in Protein

Incorporating protein-rich foods such as eggs into your breakfast has been found to be advantageous for achieving weight loss.

Replacing your typical bowl of oatmeal with a protein-enriched scramble consisting of eggs and sautéed vegetables can effectively contribute to weight loss.

Commencing the day by elevating protein intake can likewise aid in avoiding unhealthy food choices and enhancing appetite regulation throughout the day.

8. Exercise caution in consuming high-calorie beverages

Although it is widely understood, it is strongly advised to refrain from consuming milkshakes and soft drinks. However, it is worth noting that a significant number of individuals are not aware that even beverages specifically marketed as enhancing athletic performance or promoting good health can contain undesirable substances.

Beverages such as espresso, fortified waters, and sports drinks tend to have a considerably high calorie content, artificial additives, and added sugars.

Indeed, even though juice is frequently regarded as an innovative and healthful beverage, excessive consumption can lead to rapid weight gain.

Direct your focus on replenishing your body's hydration levels by consuming water in order to minimize the calorie intake throughout the course of the day.

9. Exercise Sound Judgment While Making Purchases

Creating a comprehensive shopping list and adhering to it is an excellent strategy to prevent impulsive purchases of unhealthy food items.

In addition, the act of formulating a list of items to purchase has demonstrated the potential to facilitate more nutritious dietary choices and facilitate progress towards achieving weight reduction goals.

10. Ensure Proper Hydration

Ensuring adequate hydration throughout the day is beneficial for overall well-being and can even contribute to maintaining a healthy body weight.

A study comprising a sample size of over 9,500 participants revealed that those who experienced inadequate hydration exhibited higher body mass index (BMI) values and were more prone to obesity compared to those who maintained proper hydration practices.

In addition, it has been demonstrated that individuals who consume water prior to meals tend to consume a reduced amount of calories.

11. Engage in Mindfulness While Eating

Rushing through meals or consuming food hastily can result in excessive expenditure of energy within a short span of time.

Instead, exercise mindfulness towards your food, focusing your attention on the flavors of each bite. It may result in enhanced awareness of satiety cues, reducing the likelihood of overeating (18).

Focusing on the mindful consumption of your meal, even when time is limited, can effectively mitigate excessive eating.

12. Reduce Consumption of Processed Carbohydrates

Processed carbohydrates consist of sugars and grains that have undergone removal of their fiber and other nutrients. Models encompass the utilization of refined flour, pasta, and bread.

These particular types of foods possess a low fiber content, undergo rapid processing, and only provide a short-lived sensation of satiety.

Instead, opt for sources of complex carbohydrates such as oats, ancient grains like barley and quinoa, or vegetables like potatoes and carrots.

They will assist in promoting a prolonged feeling of fullness and offer a significantly higher array of nutrients compared to processed sources of carbohydrates.

13. Increase weight resistance for effective weight reduction

Although high-impact activities such as brisk walking, jogging, and cycling are highly effective for weight loss, many individuals tend to solely focus on cardiovascular exercises and overlook the inclusion of strength training in their fitness regimens.

Incorporating resistance training into your fitness regimen can facilitate muscular development and promote overall body toning.

14. Establishing Significance-Oriented Objectives

Common motivations for individuals desiring weight loss include the desire to comfortably fit into clothing from their earlier educational years or to achieve a more favorable appearance while dressed in swimwear.

However, it is crucial to fully grasp the rationale behind your desire to lose weight and the possible positive impacts that weight loss can entail on your life. Making these objectives your foremost priority can facilitate your adherence to the plan.

Engaging in a game of tag with your children or being able to sustain activity during the entirety of a social event, such as a wedding, are examples of objectives that can help maintain your focus on achieving a positive transformation.

15. Avoid following temporary dietary trends

The prevailing trend in dietary practices is commendable for its efficacy in facilitating rapid weight loss for individuals.

However, these diets tend to be excessively restrictive and challenging to maintain. This gives rise to a cycle of intermittent dieting, wherein individuals experience temporary weight loss only to regain it afterwards.

While this pattern is common among individuals seeking expedient results, yo-yo dieting has been associated with a more notable propensity for long-term weight gain.

Additionally, studies have indicated that recurrent weight cycling can elevate the risk of developing diabetes, cardiovascular diseases, hypertension, and metabolic syndrome.

Although these diets may seem alluring, it is far wiser to opt for a practical, nutritious eating regimen that supports your body rather than depriving it.

16. Consume whole, unprocessed foods.

Maintaining precise records of the substances ingested is an exceptional approach to enhance one's well-being.

Consuming whole foods devoid of additives or preservatives ensures that you are nourishing your body with natural, nutrient-rich ingredients.

17. Formal alternative: "Form an alliance"

If you are encountering challenges in maintaining a consistent exercise routine or adhering to a healthy eating regimen, consider inviting a companion to accompany you to provide support and help you stay committed.

Research indicates that individuals who engage in weight loss and exercise programs alongside a companion exhibit increased adherence rates. In addition, they tend to experience greater weight loss compared to those who undertake the journey independently.

18. Make an effort to abstain from self-denial.

Admitting to oneself that the consumption of one's favored food items will never occur again not only appears illogical, but also has the potential to breed discontent.

Restraining oneself will only intensify the desire for the forbidden food and potentially result in indulgence upon eventual surrender.

Taking into consideration reasonable indulgences to a significant degree will demonstrate composure and hinder any potential frustration towards your newly adopted, health-conscious way of life.

19. Adopt a pragmatic approach

Drawing comparisons between oneself and models featured in magazines or prominent individuals on television not only lacks rationality but also has the potential to manifest as detrimental to one's well-being.

While possessing a strong role model can be an exceptional means of staying motivated, excessively criticizing oneself can impede progress and potentially result in unhealthy behaviors.

Consider focusing on how you feel rather than fixating on your appearance, and give centering a try. Your primary objectives should encompass the attainment of greater happiness, improved physical well-being, and enhanced health.

20. Relax and rejuvenate

Vegetables are abundant in dietary fiber and essential nutrients that your body requires.

Furthermore, augmenting your intake of vegetables can aid in promoting weight loss.

Indeed, it has been demonstrated that consuming a portion of assorted leafy greens prior to a meal can effectively induce satiety, resulting in reduced caloric intake.

21. Intelligent Eating

Indulging in unhealthy snacks has the potential to result in an increase in body weight.

A straightforward approach to facilitate weight loss or maintain a healthy body weight is to endeavor to ensure that nutritious snacks are readily available within your residence, vehicle, and workplace.

As an illustration, implementing the practice of reserving pre-portioned packs of mixed nuts in your automobile or ensuring that your refrigerator is stocked with pre-sliced vegetables accompanied by hummus can effectively aid in maintaining your discipline should a craving arise.

22. Addressing the Absence

Exhaustion may result in the pursuit of nutritionally unfavorable food choices.

Research has demonstrated that fatigue contributes to an augmentation in overall energy expenditure as it influences individuals to consume more sustenance, encompassing both nutritious and detrimental food.

Engaging in a leisurely stroll amidst nature essentially enhances one's outlook, fostering motivation and commitment towards achieving health goals.

23. Allocate a few minutes for personal reflection and self-care

Adopting a more health-conscious way of life entails prioritizing one's own well-being, even in situations where it may seem implausible.

Lifestyle frequently poses obstacles to the achievement of weight loss and wellness goals, thus it is crucial to establish a plan that incorporates dedicated personal time, and adhere to it.

Responsibilities such as employment and child-rearing hold utmost significance in life, however, prioritizing one's health should also rank among the highest priorities.

Regardless of whether this entails preparing a nutritious meal to bring to your workplace, engaging in a jog or participating in a fitness session, allocating time to prioritize self-care can have remarkable effects on both your physical and mental well-being.

24. Uncover Exercise Regimens That Bring You Genuine Pleasure

The remarkable aspect of selecting an exercise regimen resides in the boundless array of possibilities it encompasses.

Exercises that have been well-established have a greater caloric expenditure compared to alternative methods. However, it would be imprudent to select an exercise solely based on the anticipated results it may yield.

25. Support is of utmost importance.

Establishing a support system of acquaintances or family members who are invested in assisting you with your weight and wellness objectives is crucial in order to achieve successful weight reduction.

Surround yourself with individuals who possess a constructive mindset, as their influence will aid in cultivating a sustainable and health-conscious lifestyle, thereby ensuring that you remain motivated and committed to your goals.

No Convenience Foods

One of the appealing aspects of weight management programs such as Weight Watchers, South Beach, or Jenny Craig is the option to subscribe to a service that provides the convenience of having all your meals delivered to your doorstep. The portion sizes are predetermined, and the majority of the meals and snacks are either pre-prepared or can be easily heated using a microwave.

As the DASH diet is not commercially marketed, it does not offer the convenience of pre-packaged food delivery services. In addition, it is not feasible to visit the frozen food section of your nearby grocery store and access pre-cooked meals. There are no readily available smoothies or snack bars. This diet requires additional effort.

No Organized Support

Group support is also a widely embraced component found in various diet plans. Some programs provide in-person counseling, group sessions, or mentorship through peer-to-peer coaching. These attributes assist individuals in overcoming challenges during periods of reduced motivation, facilitate their ability to inquire and acquire knowledge, and gain valuable insights and expert techniques.

Although there are numerous resources available on the DASH diet, there is a lack of a structured support platform for this plan. Nonetheless, should you be contemplating the utilization of the dietary regimen, do not allow this inconvenience to impede your progress.

Any proficient registered dietitian is well-acquainted with the program, and they are equipped to assist you in formulating dietary schemes, or offer guidance and encouragement as required.

Requires Food Tracking

No calorie tracking is necessary on the DASH diet. Nonetheless, there exist prescribed calorie targets that dictate the permissible serving sizes for each food category. Therefore, you will need to select the appropriate level and make periodic adjustments as your age fluctuates or if there are any changes in your activity level. However, it is not necessary for you to monitor or tally calories.

However, adhering to the DASH diet in a meticulous manner entails the requirement to meticulously quantify portions and track the number of servings from various food groups. This procedure can be equally if not more meticulous and laborious than the practice of monitoring calorie intake.

The National Institutes of Health have made available printable versions of the DASH diet guide, which offer assistance in managing and monitoring your food intake.

With sufficient practice, the process may become more manageable. However, initially, this aspect of the program may prove daunting for certain individuals.

Primarily Intended for Purposes Other Than Facilitating Weight Reduction

While it is possible to adhere to a lower-calorie target regimen while on the DASH diet, the primary focus is not centered around achieving weight loss. Moreover, the research conducted on the DASH diet prioritizes factors other than weight reduction, instead emphasizing various health-related outcomes. It can be challenging to ascertain the comparative effectiveness of the DASH diet in relation to other dietary approaches in the context of weight loss.

The DASH diet does not incorporate a rapid weight loss phase, unlike many other weight loss programs, where individuals can quickly shed pounds to enhance their motivation and adherence to the plan. Conversely, it is probable that you will observe a gradual reduction in body weight.

Not Appropriate for Everyone

Although there exist numerous individuals who can derive advantages from adhering to the DASH diet, experts have delineated specific groups who ought to exercise prudence prior to modifying their dietary patterns to adopt this regimen.

A documented research endeavor explored the efficacy of the DASH diet among specific demographics. While scholars acknowledge the nutritional benefits of this diet for most individuals, they recommend exercising caution for patients with chronic kidney disease, chronic liver disease, and those prescribed renin-angiotensin-aldosterone system antagonists. Additionally, it is proposed that alterations to the DASH diet may be required for individuals suffering from chronic heart failure, uncontrolled type II diabetes mellitus, lactose intolerance, and celiac disease.

The report emphasizes the significance of collaborating with your healthcare provider prior to making significant alterations to your dietary or exercise regimen. They not only possess the ability to offer counsel on the potential advantages in terms of health that you might obtain, but they may also have the capacity to direct you towards a certified nutritionist or an alternate expert who can extend assistance and related provisions.

How It Compares

The DASH Diet consistently remains among the most wholesome diets accessible. Additionally, given that the guidelines for adhering to this diet are readily available at no cost and grounded in reputable academic inquiry, it is frequently endorsed by healthcare practitioners. However, there are alternative diets that are also recommended.

Delectable Morning Casserole

Ingredients:

2 minced garlic cloves
1 medium diced onion
1/2 red bell pepper, diced
Freshly ground black pepper
4 cups frozen hash browns
12 eggs
1/2 cup low fat milk
10 ounces of cooked sausage
8 ounces of shredded cheddar cheese

Directions:

To begin, generously coat the base of a crockpot with cooking spray and transfer the eggs into a spacious mixing bowl. Integrate milk with mustard, while stirring vigorously until fully amalgamated. Disperse a layer of 1/2 hash browns at the base of a crockpot, subsequently adding 1/2 portions each of sausage, garlic, onion, cheese, and bell pepper on top. Incorporate an additional stratum of hash browns, garlic, onion, sausage, cheese, and bell pepper. Proceed by evenly spreading the egg mixture over the layers and subsequently ensuring complete coverage. Next, simmer on a low heat setting for a duration of 4 and a half hours to 5 hours, or alternatively, on a high heat setting for a period of 2 to 3 hours. Please ensure that the eggs are fully cooked before they are served.

Why Does It Work?

This is a query frequently pondered by individuals, and it is a query that indeed possesses a definitive answer. The response to this inquiry is that the DASH Diet represents a nutritious dietary approach. Allow us to examine the underlying factors that contribute to the efficacy of the DASH Diet. You may find these points to be unexpected!

You experience a heightened sense of inner fulfillment, even while engaging in multiple daily eating episodes.

You experience heightened levels of energy throughout the duration of your day and seldomly encounter feelings of fatigue.

Your well-being experiences a significant improvement, both in terms of physical and mental states.

Its maintenance is facilitated by the absence of intricate regulations necessitating regular monitoring on a weekly or monthly basis.

Your discipline is commendable, as you demonstrate greater self-restraint by actively limiting your food intake through a thorough understanding of which foods to completely abstain from.

Foods to Have

The DASH Diet permits the consumption of seven distinct food categories, which encompass the following:

Vegetable

It is recommended to consume 4–5 servings of vegetables daily to maintain adherence to the DASH Diet. Vegetables possess a vast reservoir of key nutrients including magnesium, vitamins, potassium, and dietary fiber. It is important to remember to restrict your sodium consumption, however, it is advised to instead focus on the nutritional content. Selecting beans is a commendable option, albeit if you decide on canned beans, I recommend reviewing the nutritional information to ascertain the sodium content. Sweet potatoes possess a significant quantity of Vitamin A and fiber, which enhance the efficacy of blood vessels. Additional alternatives consist of winter squash, cauliflower, broccoli, spinach, carrots, kale, beetroot, garlic, onions, and tomatoes.

Fruits

Similar to vegetables, it is imperative to consume a minimum of 4–5 portions of fruit in order to avail oneself of the dietary benefits of fiber and essential energy, which contribute to optimal bodily functioning. You have the option to procure your fruits in a dried, frozen, canned, or fresh state. When purchasing canned fruits, it is advisable to carefully review the nutritional information to determine if any additional sweeteners have been incorporated. The majority of fruits serve as excellent sources of magnesium, fiber, and potassium, while simultaneously possessing minimal levels of fat. Some of the fruits that can be incorporated into the DASH Diet are apples, bananas, pears, peaches, dates, grapes, mangoes, nectarines, strawberries, blueberries, raspberries, raisins, pineapples, oranges, and melons.

Whole Grains

It is recommended that individuals consume 7-8 servings of whole grains on a daily basis in order to enhance their nutrient and fiber intake. One may contemplate a plethora of cereal options. Include pasta and bread in your diet, but refrain from garnishing them with cheesy, creamy, or buttery toppings. A selection of nutritious alternatives to consider comprises whole-grain pasta, brown rice, air-popped popcorn, whole oats, quinoa, and whole-grain bread.

Dairy Products

When making the selection of dairy products to incorporate into your diet, it is important to take into account both low-fat and fat-free options. These items serve as a reliable and beneficial source of essential nutrients such as vitamin D, calcium, and protein. One may choose between a serving of yogurt or milk, or opt for a portion of cheese weighing 1.5 ounces. Alternative choices consist of milk that is low in fat content, such as skim milk or fat-free milk, as well as cheese that is low in fat or completely fat-free, and yogurt that is low in fat or completely fat-free. Given their lack of dairy properties, it is essential to note that coconut and almond milk cannot be considered as viable substitutes for dairy-based products. Milk encompasses vital nutrients necessary for the assimilation of potassium, calcium, and vitamin D.

Lean Protein

When adhering to the DASH Diet, it is recommended to consume a minimum of six servings of poultry, lean meat, or fish per day. Lean and skinless meat are highly commendable sources of essential nutrients such as vitamin B complex, zinc, iron, and protein. A selection of options worth contemplating encompasses seafood and fish, which provide a source of Omega 3 fatty acids and contribute to the reduction of cholesterol levels. Nevertheless, it is advisable to opt for freshly prepared food rather than canned options in order to minimize the consumption of sodium and preservatives. You have the option to employ baking, grilling, or roasting methods, while refraining from utilizing frying. Additional alternatives include individual servings of eggs and skinless lean poultry (it is advised to always remove the skin).

Edible legumes and seeds

When formulating a weekly dietary schedule, it is important to incorporate 5–6 portions of beans, legumes, nuts, and seeds. These foods serve as an excellent dietary source of magnesium, phytochemicals, protein, and fiber. Given that the majority of these options are calorie-dense, it is imperative that you remain mindful of your intake. A unitary portion could consist of 2 tablespoons of nuts. Pistachios, lentils, kidney beans, peas, cashews, peanuts, almonds, and various other food items constitute a selection of commonly found edibles within this particular category.

Lipids and Hydrocarbons

As per the guidance of nutrition experts, it is recommended to incorporate 2-3 servings of fats and oils in your daily diet. These factors are vital for the enhancement of the immune system and the absorption of nutrients. However, it is important to exercise prudence and regulate the quantity you utilize, as unmanaged consumption of abundant fats and oils can lead to obesity, the development of diabetes, and cardiovascular ailments. A possible rephrasing in a formal tone could be: A single portion may consist of either a teaspoon of mayonnaise or a tablespoon of salad dressing, soft margarine, or vegetable oil. Additional alternatives consist of coconut oil, extra virgin olive oil, and peanuts.

Sucrose and Confections

Indeed, the DASH Diet prescribes a cap of no more than five servings of sugar per week, representing a delightful surprise for adherents. This plan permits moderate indulgence in sweet treats. Nonetheless, it is essential to strive for options that have a lesser proportion of fat. An excellent selection of items that constitute a serving include jelly beans, oatmeal cookies or bars with reduced fat content, or fruit sorbet. Various options for sweeteners that you may contemplate consist of sugar, unprocessed honey, agave syrup, and maple syrup. The majority of these are predominantly comprised of natural sweeteners, making them a favorable option.

Recommended Dietary Restrictions for Optimal Compliance with the DASH Diet

While we have previously covered various foods that should be avoided, we have decided to compile them here for ease of reference. There are no food items pertaining to fruits and vegetables that are deemed forbidden. Let us commence with the first topic of discussion, namely grains.

Prohibited Grains

White bread.

White rice.

White pasta.

White, refined flour.

White bread rolls for hamburgers and hot dogs.

Sourdough bread.

French bread.

Any cereal containing additional sugar.

Refined grains and flour-based breakfast cereals.

Any snacks containing sugar.

Any snacks with elevated sodium levels (for instance, Triscuits, despite being whole grain, possess a substantial amount of salt.) Acquire a low sodium alternative.

Snacks that incorporate trans fats.

Dairy

Furthermore, let us now shift our attention towards the dairy section. From a technical standpoint, it is imperative to only partake in low-fat options when consuming milk, yogurt, and cheese. Nevertheless, as previously stated, research indicates that there is no significant disparity in outcomes when consuming whole-fat varieties, and in certain individuals, it may even yield superior results.

Nevertheless, certain dairy products ought to be avoided: "

Butter and ghee.

Heavy cream.

Whipped cream.

Half-and-Half.

Buttermilk.

Egg nog.

Aggregate Caloric Requirements Across Diverse Individuals Considering Factors Of Age, Gender, And Body Mass

If your objective is to reduce body weight, it is advisable to familiarize yourself with the caloric quantities applicable to individuals, accounting for various factors. In order to achieve this, we have meticulously assembled this comprehensive table containing detailed calorie values corresponding to different profiles of gender, age, and weight. Kindly be informed that the aforementioned figures should be regarded as approximate calculations, as they have been derived from respective averages obtained from distinguished sources such as The World Health Organization and the International Society of Sports Nutrition International Journal of Sports Nutrition and Exercise

Metabolism. The numerical values might vary slightly based on additional factors, including the individual's level of physical activity or their geographical circumstance.

The male and female averages presented herein do not encompass individuals in the younger age groups, as the Food and Agriculture Organization of the United Nations has released updated estimates for this specific demographic in January 2016. Nevertheless, it is pertinent to note that the aforementioned data can still be employed as an influential factor, as the weight distribution within these cohorts generally demonstrates relative stability throughout their lifespan.

According to the presented data, it seems evident that the average caloric demand decreases in both males and females as they grow older, reaching a decline during middle age. Subsequently, a gradual upturn commences in individuals aged in their 60s and 70s of both genders. This can be attributed to factors such as a decline in physical activity levels, a natural outcome that accompanies the aging process. Male individuals who have reached the age of 66 require an approximate daily caloric intake ranging from 2,400 to 3,200 calories, whereas women in the same age bracket necessitate an estimated daily caloric intake of 2,000 to 2,400 calories.

It is essential to recognize the distinctions between these figures and the suggested daily caloric intake of 2,000 per day, as proposed by numerous weight loss programs for a variety of reasons. The disparity in these figures arises from the fact that they are mean values derived from an elderly cohort, without factoring in individual circumstances such as levels of physical activity or medical considerations.

Commencing With The Dash Diet

What are the methods I can employ to incorporate Dash into my daily routine?

This dietary regimen should adhere to a reduced calorie content, limited sodium intake (restricted salt consumption), minimal fat consumption, low sugar consumption, and exclude red meat.

However, it is essential that it comprises whole grains, fruits, vegetables, and legumes. Low-fat dairy products encompass fish, poultry, and lean meat.

It is advisable to occasionally incorporate certain types of nuts and seeds into one's diet. While the intention is to reduce the consumption of red meat, it is acceptable for them to partake in it occasionally.

There exist a multitude of uncomplicated guidelines that individuals of all backgrounds can gradually adopt in order to initiate the adoption of healthier dietary habits within the framework of the DASH diet.

The following are alternative expressions in a more formal tone: "Presented below are a few examples:"

• Increase the quantity of vegetables on the plate by twofold. The optimal choice is to acquire vegetables that are freshly obtained from the market.

- Incorporate fruits into your muesli. - Add fruits to your muesli mixture. - Introduce fruit to your muesli for added flavor and nutrition. - Enhance your muesli by including a variety of fresh fruits. - Include fruits as a complementary ingredient in your muesli. These may include raspberries, blueberries, or bananas. Furthermore, in relation to cereals, oats are recommended.

• Opt for a fat-free unsweetened yogurt and incorporate freshly cut fruits for a delightful fruit yogurt devoid of added sugars. They present an intriguing choice and are replete with essential vitamins.

• Prepare homemade smoothies: The DASH diet permits the consumption of smoothies as long as they do not contain any additional sugar. Should you opt to incorporate milk into your preparation, it is imperative that it be of low-fat content and comprise of freshly sourced fruits. The optimal approach would be to purchase vegetables that are either freshly sourced or available in frozen form, conveniently pre-cut and prepared for consumption.

• The examples provided include broccoli, carrots, lettuce, and cauliflower. The DASH diet also underscores the significance of dishes that are more vibrant in color, as they are deemed superior.

Grain:

Consume 6 to 8 servings per day.

This encompasses various food items such as bread, cereal, rice, and pasta. A daily portion of bread along with a serving of rice or pasta would be acceptable. It is advisable to opt for cereals made from whole grain. This particular item possesses a higher content of dietary fiber. Please select either pasta, bread, or brown rice as your preferred option for the grain component.

Vegetables:

Consumption of 4 to 5 servings on a daily basis is recommended.

Vegetables possess inherent properties of abundant dietary fiber, essential nutrients, and valuable vitamins. Vegetables such as tomatoes, carrots, and green vegetables like broccoli possess a significant abundance of essential minerals such as potassium and magnesium.

Consider a portion to be equivalent to a modest serving of lettuce or half of a portion of carrots.

Fruit:

Consumption of four to five servings per day is recommended.

Similar to vegetables, fruits are likewise abundant in dietary fiber, vitamins, and minerals.

Thus, the fruit is well-suited as a morning or post-lunch refreshment or after-dinner treat.

Dairy products:

Consumption of 2 to 3 servings per day is recommended.

They serve as a reliable source of calcium, vitamin D, and protein.

It is imperative to select dairy products that are low in fat. For instance, an illustration of a low-fat dairy item could be a serving of skim milk accompanied by a skim milk-based yogurt. Frozen yogurt is exceptionally well-suited for a dessert, as it can be elevated with the addition of fresh fruit.

"White meat, poultry, and seafood:

A limit of 6 servings per day.

Meat serves as a valuable reservoir of protein, in addition to being a rich source of group B vitamins, iron, and zinc.

The removal of chicken skin is recommended due to its elevated fat content.

Give preference to fish varieties that possess abundant omega-3 fatty acids.

"Assortment of non-shell tree seeds and edible pulses:

Four to five servings per week

Almonds, sunflower or pumpkin seeds, legumes, and lentils are abundant sources of magnesium, potassium, protein, and dietary fiber.

Tofu can serve as an excellent substitute for meat; however, it is important to acknowledge that soy, particularly the sauce, contains high levels of sodium and therefore should be abstained from.

Lipids and hydrocarbons:

It is recommended to consume 2 to 3 servings per day.

It is advisable to restrict the consumption of fats and oils due to their high caloric content. It is recommended to restrict the consumption of these types of fats to less than 30% of the daily calorie intake.

It is imperative to abstain from the consumption of saturated fats. It is imperative to steer clear of industrial foods and pastries under any circumstances.

Sweets:

Limit consumption to no more than one serving per day.

Incorporating a small quantity of jam into one's breakfast or adding a teaspoon of sugar to the coffee adequately meets the requirement for a single serving.

What are the prohibited foods in the DASH Diet?

• Beef

• Bacon

• Lamb

• Margarine

• Deep-fried cuisine • Foods that are cooked by immersing in hot oil • Dishes prepared through frying in oil or fat • Cuisine that undergoes the process of deep-frying

• Plant-based fat

• Lard

All the protein must possess low fat content. Therefore, adhere to selecting white meat, turkey meat, and fish during your shopping endeavors. Additional viable sources of protein may include low-fat yogurt and legumes.

Potassium: A Valuable Ally

In the preceding segments of this book, we have diligently emphasized the efficacy of fruits, vegetables, and organic food items.

There exists a rationale behind this occurrence. Across all levels of biological organization, including the cellular level, adopting a more nutritious dietary pattern yields significant and transformative effects. By consuming unprocessed foods, individuals can enhance their nutrient intake and address the widespread lack of essential nutrients, such as potassium, which is prevalent among the majority of Americans.

Fundamentally, potassium serves as a catalyst for optimal physiological performance within the human body.

The human body requires potassium in order to regulate renal function and facilitate the proper functioning of nerves and muscles. Insufficient intake of potassium may lead to hypertension, calcium depletion in bone structure, and the formation of renal calculi (National Institutes of Health, n.d.). Individuals who experience inadequate potassium intake are also at an elevated risk of developing stroke, coronary heart disease, hypertension, and type 2 diabetes.

Furthermore, potassium assists in the regulation of sodium levels within the body, thereby mitigating certain detrimental impacts, as elaborated upon in Chapter 1. At a molecular level, cellular functioning is accomplished through the exchange of sodium and potassium ions across the intracellular and extracellular membranes. In essence, the optimization of cellular function and overall bodily performance can be achieved by elevating potassium consumption and reducing sodium levels. Fortunately, fruits and vegetables, which occupy a central position in the DASH diet, inherently possess abundant amounts of potassium. Bananas are primarily renowned for their high potassium content, closely accompanied by sweet potatoes. These two ingredients have been extensively integrated into our repertoire of recipes. In addition to the aforementioned items, it is worth noting that lentils, nuts, soybeans, kidney beans, leafy greens, nonfat milk, and yogurt also serve as noteworthy sources of potassium.

While ensuring an ample supply of these ingredients is crucial, it is equally imperative to acquire knowledge and discernment in order to make optimal selections in both grocery stores and dining establishments. Although the most reliable method of protecting against excessive sodium consumption is through the preparation of one's own meals and meticulous ingredient selection, this approach may not always be feasible. The following pages will encompass recommendations and strategies to enhance the efficiency of your shopping cart or facilitate your takeaway order.

Eating Out

As consumers exert increased pressure on restaurant chains to incorporate healthier ingredients and enhance transparency regarding their food preparation, the availability of more nutritious options is progressively improving. If you possess prior knowledge of the restaurant you intend to visit, it would be prudent to conduct thorough research in advance. Restaurant websites are progressively incorporating nutritional details for individual menu items, and a subset of restaurants will willingly furnish an elaborate nutritional fact sheet upon request.

Effective communication is crucial to ensuring a satisfactory dining experience. Inquire with the server as to whether there are any menu options specifically denoted as low in sodium or suitable for individuals seeking heart-healthy alternatives. Additionally, it may be possible for you to make a formal request to the chefs, asking them to refrain from including any additional salt in their culinary preparations. In the absence of any other options, it is advisable to select dishes that are prepared by baking rather than frying or coating with batter. Furthermore, whenever feasible, it is recommended to replace starchy items with vegetables or fruits. In order to maintain control over the size of your portions, there are two options available: either divide your meals into smaller portions or request a container in advance to package a portion of the meal for consumption on a subsequent day.

SHOPPING

We are currently witnessing a greater assortment of products in grocery establishments compared to previous years. Invariably, items that are not readily obtainable in a state of freshness can be acquired in the form of preserved, frozen, or synthetic alternatives. We would strongly advise the purchase of fresh ingredients and the proactive preparation of as many items as feasible beforehand.

Nevertheless, in instances where time is limited and the extent of your preparation tasks is extensive, you may find it necessary to purchase food that contains preservatives.

If feasible, undertake some preliminary research on the spectrums of sodium levels that you encounter whilst perambulating each aisle. You might observe that certain brands employ a higher sodium content in the packaging of their products compared to other brands. While browsing for frozen fruits or vegetables, it is advisable to inspect the packaging for the phrase "fresh frozen" as such products are typically processed with minimal use of preservatives. One could reduce the sodium content in canned or frozen produce by rinsing and draining the ingredients before incorporating them into your culinary preparations. It is advised to consistently choose fresh fruits and vegetables as a preference over frozen or canned options whenever feasible. In an ideal scenario, the usually designated area in your freezer for storing packaged goods can now be repurposed as a space to conveniently preserve nutritious meals for busy individuals.

In a like manner, abstain from utilizing salt-infused mixtures that contain excessive levels of sodium. Seasonings, such as those containing garlic and onion salt, can be readily replaced with onion powder and garlic powder. Engage in the endeavor of crafting your own unique combinations of spices, like those inspired by Italian or Mediterranean culinary traditions. Please be aware that a measurement of 1-½ tsp of salt corresponds to the recommended daily intake of sodium. Alternatively, it can be observed that this culinary guide extensively incorporates a variety of herbs and spices, such as oregano, cilantro, basil, thyme, cumin, cinnamon, allspice, cloves, and paprika. When selecting condiments, it is advisable to seek labels that indicate the absence of salt, reduced sodium content, or complete absence of sodium.

Contemplate replacing high-fat meat choices with protein sources that are lower in fat content, or alternatively, omitting meat altogether from one's diet. Three ounces of poultry or fish can contain a maximum of 90 mg of naturally-occurring sodium, whereas lean roasted ham can contain as much as 1,020 mg per serving. We have incorporated a selection of vegetarian and vegan recipes to foster the concept that meat is not an indispensable component of every dish. If executed properly, one can obtain the necessary protein and fat without the consumption of any kind of meat.

Lastly, endeavor to procure an abundant supply of non-perishable goods that are consistently mentioned throughout the contents of this literary work. Numerous ingredients will serve a useful purpose in various recipes, and opting for bulk purchases could demonstrate greater cost-effectiveness. In this book, there is a strong reliance on several key ingredients such as brown rice, basmati rice, apple cider vinegar, black beans, kidney beans, fresh frozen berries, tahini, lime juice, lemon juice, and balsamic vinegar.

Construct Your Culinary Arsenal

The items you purchase for your daily meals hold the same level of utility as the utensils you bring into the kitchen. It is likely that you will have to allocate a greater amount of time to the activity of cooking and food preparation than you are accustomed to. This implies that you may embark on a shopping excursion. We have incorporated in this book designs that are relatively attainable. Nevertheless, for the sake of clarity and shared understanding, provided below is a compilation of guidelines that could aid you in your endeavor as both a culinary practitioner and a dedicated follower of the DASH diet:

• Culinary Tool: Within the vast array of cutting equipment accessible to culinary enthusiasts, only a handful compare in efficacy to a well-honed chef's knife. This particular utensil is highly effective for the purpose of cutting a wide range of items, with a particular emphasis on vegetables. Please rest assured that there is no need to be concerned about purchasing a knife of professional quality or acquiring a new one if you currently possess one. This knife possesses the capability to facilitate a precise and uniform cutting experience.

- Crock-Pot: Crock-Pots symbolize the uncelebrated champions of the corporate day. Few sensations are more delightful than effortlessly placing your ingredients into the cooking vessel, allowing it to simmer overnight or throughout the workday, and rediscovering a delectable, succulent meal waiting for you at day's end. The passage of time and the presence of an airtight environment facilitate the infusion of flavors, herbs, and spices into various selections of meat, main courses, and similar dishes. Certain individuals even choose to integrate several slow cookers of varying sizes in order to enhance the efficiency of their cooking process. Slow cookers are available at an affordable starting price of $20, a notable advantage when taking into account the high quality of the final outcome.

• Frying pan: The majority of main courses commonly commence and culminate by being prepared in a frying pan. This item proves to be particularly useful, especially in the context of breakfast-related items. This cooking tool is suitable for preparing vegetables including onions and peppers, using the heart-healthy option of olive oil.

• Saucepan: This utensil proves to be highly handy for the purpose of amalgamating ingredients that do not necessitate excessive attention. Many paellas and stir fry-inspired dishes may require you to utilize your practical saucepan.

• Basting brush: Enhance the flavors and maximize the utility of your exquisite sauces and spice concoctions by investing in a superior basting brush.

This paintbrush-shaped tool proves to be quite useful for applying the finishing touches to a marinade or for delicately coating ingredients prior to presentation.

• Stockpot: Stockpots serve as indispensable tools for preparing generously portioned meals that cater to a large number of individuals, making them an essential component for the soup recipes contained within this cookbook. This spacious receptacle provides assurance in preventing any spillage caused by excessive boiling.

• Food Processor: In many instances, blenders and food processors can be employed concurrently. This assertion may not hold true in the context of this particular cookbook. The variances may appear minute, yet they are of immense significance when it comes to the culinary preparations outlined within this book. Blenders are commonly employed in the production of liquid concoctions. Food processors are utilized for the purpose of combining and shredding desiccated components. Food processors play a crucial role in finely pulverizing challenging ingredients, which would otherwise pose difficulties in terms of chopping, such as nuts for garnishing or tomatoes for making salsa. Spare yourself the anguish of the realization that the task of finely chopping hazelnuts for a cream solution cannot be accomplished successfully through the utilization of an inexpensive food processor.

Avocado Spinach Salad

Ingredients:

- 1 ripe avocado
- NASTURTIUMS
- Salt pepper
- 150g spinach leaves
- ½ LEMON
- 1 tablespoon elderflower syrup
- 1 tablespoon sesame oil

Preparation:

Thoroughly cleanse and rinse the spinach with care. Incorporate approximately 2 tablespoons of the lemon juice, together with the elderflower syrup and sesame oil, into the salad dressing mixture while gently stirring. Add salt and pepper to taste. Carefully peel and thinly slice the avocado, subsequently integrating them with the sauce. Incorporate the spinach into the mixture and embellish with the cress.

Canned Salmon

Ingredient

- 1 can of salmon, drained and flaked
- 1/4 cup of mild pickled pepper rings, chopped
- 1/4 cup of mayo
- 1 tbsp of pepper juice, pickled

Instructions

Mix mayo, peppers, salmon, & pepper juice into a bowl.
Serve and enjoy.

While the desire for a more slender waistline and improved health may understandably lead you to choose the DASH diet, it is important to note that there are additional factors to consider when contemplating the adoption of this dietary approach. The items encompassed are as follows:

Weight Loss

DASH promotes significantly lower fat intake compared to the typical American diet. This implies that it possesses a reduced caloric content. This dietary regimen excludes and diminishes the consumption of unhealthy fats, fast food, fried foods, and highly processed food items. On the contrary, it places emphasis on health-enhancing fats such as saturated fats and beneficial saturated fats like omega-3 fats, which confer positive effects on the body and facilitate weight reduction. These are predominantly found in food items that have reduced calorie content. The substantial presence of dietary fiber in the majority of the food items endorsed by the DASH diet represents an additional significant factor in promoting weight reduction. Consumption of fibers facilitates a sensation of fullness while concurrently supporting the digestive process, enabling the body to expel waste materials and impeding the rapid assimilation of sugars and fats. It facilitates proficient management and responsiveness to insulin, in contrast to the potential hazards and manifestations of metabolic syndrome.

The substantial uptake or utilization of fresh vegetables and fruits corresponds to elevated levels of vitamin C and antioxidants. Vitamin C plays a crucial role in mitigating stress by reducing the synthesis of the stress hormone, cortisol. This hormone also governs the accumulation of adipose tissue in the abdominal region. Consequently, the food you consume will not be stored as adipose tissue in your abdominal region. Furthermore, vitamin C plays a pivotal role in the facilitation of fat transportation by serving as a fundamental component of L-carnitine. When the body is signaled or prompted that the fat is no longer necessary, it undergoes a transformation into glucose which can be utilized as a source of energy. The human body necessitates adequate levels of vitamin C in order to produce L-carnitine endogenously. This implies that it is essential to incorporate the daily intake of vitamin C into one's diet in order to facilitate weight loss, as vitamin C primarily functions to combat infection and repair compromised cells.

The DASH diet also promotes individualized caloric intake, taking into account factors such as weight loss objectives, existing weight, body composition, and level of physical activity. This dietary approach refrains from ingesting an inadequate amount of calories, which may result in the undesirable loss of muscle mass rather than fat, all the while ensuring adequate nutrient intake to sustain your activity level.

Heart Disease

Individuals presenting with a concurrent occurrence of hypertension, metabolic syndrome, and type 2 diabetes are predisposed to develop cardiovascular disease. The DASH diet's comprehensive approach to these conditions indicates its potential to enhance the body's resilience against heart disease. This diet possesses excellent attributes, even in the absence of pre-existing conditions. Cardiovascular disease accounts for the highest mortality rate among the American population. Healthcare professionals advise consuming a diet that is low in detrimental fats and rich in beneficial fats, and the inclusion of fiber in your diet will have a favorable impact on the health of your heart. The American Heart Association advocates for the adoption of the DASH diet due to its positive impact on heart health. In addition to bolstering cardiovascular well-being, this dietary regimen exerts a favorable impact on the colon and gastrointestinal tract.

Metabolic Syndrome

The phrase metabolic syndrome is employed to describe a cluster of symptoms correlated with insulin resistance and obesity. This condition is occasionally referred to as pre-diabetes due to its potential progression into type 2 diabetes when left uncontrolled. Certain indicators commonly associated with metabolic syndrome include elevated blood glucose levels, increased abdominal circumference, raised levels of high-density lipoprotein (HDL), and elevated levels of triglycerides. The primary objective of the DASH diet is to counteract these undesirable symptoms. The DASH diet encompasses a reduction in the intake of unhealthy fats, coupled with an elevation in the consumption of beneficial fats and dietary fiber, with the intention of diminishing triglyceride and HDL cholesterol levels. The nutrients derived from adhering to the DASH diet, in conjunction with the possible reduction of abdominal fat, work to mitigate the effects of metabolic syndrome, thereby facilitating an optimal state of health.

Type 2 Diabetes

According to the U.S. News and World Report, the DASH diet has been recognized as the most effective dietary approach in managing type 2 diabetes and mitigating the chances of developing diabetes. The rationale for this is straightforward. The foods integrated into the DASH diet facilitate the enhancement of the health of individuals afflicted with diabetes. For example, nuts serve to regulate glucose levels in individuals diagnosed with diabetes. Concurrently, the presence of a substantial amount of dietary fiber will decelerate the rate of sugar absorption, thereby contributing to the stabilization of blood glucose levels. The assortment of vegetables and fruits included in the DASH diet are abundant in antioxidants, which aid in mitigating complications associated with type 2 diabetes. The DASH diet has the potential to exert a beneficial impact on individuals with type 2 diabetes, primarily through the facilitation of weight reduction, particularly targeting visceral adipose tissue, which is closely linked with insulin resistance.

Controlled Blood Pressure

The principal advantage of the DASH diet and the rationale behind its endorsement by nutritionists and physicians lie in its remarkable benefits. Adhering to the DASH diet facilitates the maintenance of optimal blood pressure levels. This dietary plan is highly suitable for individuals who are currently under medication for blood pressure regulation, as well as those who exhibit prehypertension indications and desire more effective strategies for symptom management. The DASH program has been specifically formulated to assist in managing hypertension and has been substantiated through rigorous scientific research.

Healthy Eating

Let's face it. One of the factors contributing to the prevalence of high blood pressure among the majority of individuals is the correlation between excessive weight or obesity and suboptimal dietary choices. Adopting the DASH diet facilitates a transformation towards a nutritious eating regimen, allowing for sustained improvements in health and well-being. Consequently, you will allocate a greater amount of time in the culinary space, engaged in the preparation of nourishing meals rather than resorting to conveniently accessible processed alternatives. Furthermore, you will derive immense pleasure during your meal sessions as your plate will be abundantly adorned with nutrient-rich sustenance. DASH additionally encourages the exploration of unfamiliar vegetables and fruits, as well as the utilization of salt-free seasonings, allowing for the creation of appetizing dishes that broaden your culinary horizons.

Impacts on the Susceptibility to Osteoporosis

Most strategies for preventing and managing osteoporosis involve augmenting your consumption of calcium and vitamin D, nutrients prevalent in the recommended foods of the DASH diet. When combined with a decreased consumption of sodium, it serves as evidence that the DASH diet is highly advantageous for the maintenance of bone health. Certain research studies have yielded compelling evidence indicating a considerable decrease in bone remodeling among individuals who adhered to the Dietary Approaches to Stop Hypertension (DASH) diet. When administered consistently for a prolonged duration, the DASH diet is shown to enhance bone mineral status. Additional nutrients, exhibiting ample presence within the DASH diet, that contribute favorably to the maintenance of long-term bone health encompass vitamin C, antioxidants, magnesium, and polyphenols.

Healthy Cholesterol Levels

As the majority of the fruits, beans, nuts, whole grains, and vegetables suggested within the framework of the DASH diet possess abundant dietary fiber, these options can be consumed in conjunction with fish and lean meat, while concurrently moderating the consumption of refined carbohydrates and confectionery items. It significantly contributes to the enhancement of your cholesterol profile.

Healthier Kidneys

The DASH diet is advised for maintaining kidney health due to the generous quantities of magnesium, potassium, calcium, and dietary fiber found in the suggested food choices. The emphasis on lowering sodium consumption also offers a benefit in the event of potential kidney disease. However, it is advisable to limit the implementation of the DASH diet solely to individuals with chronic kidney disease and those receiving dialysis, unless they are carefully supervised by experienced healthcare professionals.

Impact on Select Types of Cancer

Scientists have conducted investigations on the correlation between the DASH diet and specific forms of cancer, and have discovered a favorable link which pertains to the mitigation of salt consumption and the vigilance in monitoring dietary fat intake. The diet's association with various forms of cancer such as rectal, colon, esophageal, pulmonary, gastric, renal, and prostatic is due to its diminished intake of red substances. Consuming ample amounts of fresh produce aids in reducing the risk of developing different types of cancers, while promoting the inclusion of low-fat dairy products enhances the overall health of the colon.

Improved mental well-being Enhanced psychological state

The DASH diet has the potential to enhance one's mood by mitigating the symptoms of mental health conditions such as anxiety or depression. It is linked to several lifestyle modifications, encompassing the avoidance of tobacco, the moderation of alcohol consumption, and the consistent participation in physical exercise. Furthermore, the incorporation of nourishing foods into one's dietary intake also aids in equilibrating hormones and chemicals in the brain and body, subsequently leading to enhanced mental well-being and overall physical health.

Anti-Aging Properties

Numerous individuals who adhere to the DASH diet have affirmed the notion that this dietary regimen aids in mitigating certain manifestations of the aging process, thereby facilitating a more youthful appearance and overall vitality. Enhancing your intake of fresh produce abundant in antioxidants will facilitate the regeneration of your hair and skin, invigorate and fortify your joints, muscles, and bones, promote weight loss, and foster an improved sense of well-being.

www.ingramcontent.com/pod-product-compliance
Lightning Source LLC
Chambersburg PA
CBHW051737020426
42333CB00014B/1360